YOU ARE BEAUTIFUL

ERIC REESE

ISBN: 978-1-925988-50-5

CONTENTS

We live in a society that places a high degree of importance on physical appearance. Television, movies, magazines and billboards all display attractive people. We see men and women (more women) running to plastic surgeons, having many different kinds of procedures done simply to enhance their appearance. Our society is obsessed with physical beauty, and many women are caught up in that obsession as well.

But should beauty really be that important

for a woman? Is beauty something that a woman should strive for? What makes a woman truly beautiful?

A woman can and should be beautiful—God designed her to be that way. Her skin, hair and other features were created to be soft and appealing, and her body was fashioned to be attractive and beautiful to men. A woman was designed to be attractive, and most women want to be beautiful. However, the physical side of beauty is just a small part of what makes a woman truly beautiful.

Our society places a high emphasis on the physical aspect of beauty and neglects the other elements that really make a woman totally beautiful. A beautiful woman is not just physically appealing; she is appealing in many different areas. Because our society so largely emphasizes the physical nature of beauty, you want to explore with you all of the areas that make up true beauty and bring out the missing dimension in beauty.

CHAPTER ONE

OUTER BEAUTY

A truly beautiful woman is physically appealing. Not all women are gifted with perfection of physical features, but fortunately, this is not the only prerequisite for beauty. Women tend to take a critical look at their individual features and flaws and feel this is what makes them attractive or not, whereas a man tends to look at the overall impression a woman creates. What a woman does with what she has is very important in making herself attractive.

Physical beauty is really within the reach of any woman.

The most influential factor in a woman's physical beauty is her health. When a woman is healthy, she has an attractive glow about her. Good health adds more color to the face and skin and helps produce more energy. A balanced, nutritious diet and exercise plan will help a woman to have this healthy glow. It will also help to keep excess weight off and produce a more attractive physique. When a woman is striving to follow the health laws she looks and feels more beautiful.

Another key factor of womanly beauty is looking feminine. A woman should look like a woman, not a man. A woman can achieve this through her dress and hairstyle.

CHAPTER TWO

INNER BEAUTY

A beautiful woman is not only admired for her physical appearance; she is admired for her inner qualities as well. There are many inner qualities that make a woman beautiful.

CHAPTER THREE

NATURAL BEAUTY TIPS FOR WOMEN

If you are a college going person or a working woman, these natural homemade beauty tips for women are helpful for every woman. Beauty brands come up with the new products every day and sometimes it's so confusing. We am not here to slam the beauty brands because we do use some of the beauty products but most of them sell fake promises.They attract people through fancy advertisements. How can a customer be smart and not get confused. It's quite not possible.

With the help of some natural homemade beauty tips, you are going to get the best results. If you personally use all these homemade remedies and trust me it really works. Market products give you the instant results but these results last for a short period of time. If you want to see the difference in your skin, you have to be patient and consistent. Below are the most effective and natural homemade beauty tips for women.

Natural homemade beauty tips for women:

1. For dry skin: If you live in a humid weather, your skin becomes really dry and specially when you have dry skin type. Your skin lacks moisture. You need moisture in your skin to make it look soft and supple. Take two tablespoons of milk and add honey in it. Take a

cotton ball and apply this mixture on your face. Apply it at night and keep it for 30 minutes and wash your face with the cold water.

2. For oily skin: This skin type is really complicated and we often suffer from the blackheads and the whiteheads and the stubborn pimples. The skin produces excess of sebum and the sebum gets blocked in the pores thus resulting in pimples. The oily skin also needs to be moisturized. When the skin becomes too dry, it produces excess oil. You need to keep your skin clean and clear. You can use oatmeal mask, Take some oatmeal and add honey in it. Apply this mask for 30 minutes and wash it off with the cold water. Your skin will feel fresh.

3. For blackheads: When the skin is

exposed to the dirt and pollution, the dirt gets deposited in the pores and results in the blackheads. These blackheads are very stubborn. You can use this natural homemade beauty tip to get rid of the dirt. Take an egg white and add honey and lemon in it. Apply this all over your face and leave it for 20-30 minutes. To get rid of the blackheads on the nose, Take one tablespoon of baking powder and add some lemon in it. Now apply this on your nose and leave it for 30 minutes. It is going to irritate for a while but it;s natural. It works like a miracle and your skin will look so clear.

4. For instant glowing skin: Use this natural homemade beauty tip to get an instant glowing skin. Take some honey and add few drops of lemon in it. Now apply this mask on you

face and wash it with the cold water after 30 minutes.

5. For dark circles: We are living in a busy world under so much work pressure and stress. Lack of sleep and exposure to the gadgets for a long time leads to the stubborn dark circles under the eyes. Take some almond oil and massage the under eye area with this oil clockwise and anti clockwise. You can take some raw milk and add few drops of rose water in it. Apply this mixture with the help of a cotton ball. You can leave this overnight and wash it with the help of cold water in the morning.

6. For skin lightening: If your skin is exposed to the sun, it can tan quickly. Potato juice helps in lightening the skin.

7. For fresh dewy skin. Cut some

cucumbers and soak it in the water overnight. Now wash you face with this water early in the morning. Your skin will look instantly fresh and dewy.

8. For moisturizing skin: Wash your face with the honey and often skip the cleanser in the morning and wash your face just with the honey. It makes my skin very soft and maintains the PH balance of the skin.

9. For pimples and acne: You can use a face pack of multani mitti and rose water once in a week to get rid of the dirt. Add some honey or few drops of coconut oil if you have extra dry skin. Apply this pack for 20 minutes and wash your face with the cold water.

10. For facial hair: Hormonal changes can lead to the facial growth. When

there is a fluctuation in your hormones, it disturbs the balance and leads to the growth of hair on the chin and jawline areas. You can use a face pack made with besan (gram flour) sugar and lemon. Apply this pack for 20 minutes and wash it off with the cold water. Use this pack twice a week to see the faster results. It does not remove all the hair but gradually lightens the hair and growth.

These were some highly effective and natural homemade beauty tips for women.

Use these natural homemade beauty tips and have seen a great change in the quality of your skin. You need to make sure that you are taking a healthy diet because at the end, no matter what you apply outside, if you don't take care of your diet, it won't make any difference. You need to eat the right food. Patience is the key. Don't expect the instant miracles. Who ever promises you an instant result are sure to offer the fake products. Having a healthy and great skin takes a lot of time and extra efforts unless you are born with it naturally.

CHAPTER FOUR

BEAUTY AND DYNAMIC

Beauty is only skin deep' and in one sense it is only skin deep if you view the top layer, the first look see, a glimpse of the outer or the first impression of what you initially see from a place of ego, illusion and being relatively asleep to truth. On the other hand, beauty is transparent, luminous shining vitality and is other worldly when you see it from a place of deep truth as it expresses itself through twinkling eyes, soft healthy skin and shiny hair that all share the secret of true beauty - that which cannot be touched by any cream, scalpel or tingling burning itchy treatment that all promise endless youthful beauty. Beauty is an attitude, a confidence, an inner knowing of secrets for timeless and ageless living, with grace and appreciation as our dearest companions. Grace and appreciation for every human experience we have from early childhood, through the growing pains of adolescence ~ to the freedom and exploration of our twenties - to the choices of family, career and the myriad of responsibilities that dot our thirties, forties and onwards to the freedom once again of letting go of all that we thought we were and reinventing ourselves so the decades of the fifties, sixties and beyond can allow wisdom and childhood innocence one again to play together and light the way for the ones coming up behind. I've discovered three little secrets for true luminous beauty and I'm excited to share them with you!

The Secret comes as no surprise it can be difficult to respect and resolve to make a life long habit. It's simply getting a good night's sleep, night after night, month after month, year after year for the duration of your life. Of course they'll be nights were you lay awake wondering, worrying, plotting, planning, wishing and whiling away the hours as your hormones get the better of you, so I'm referring to the majority of nights throughout your life. Making it a priority in your life of setting the stage, the room, the routine and the atmosphere to ensure a good night's sleep because you're in the know about the secret benefits of habitual deeply restorative, regenerative and rejuvenating nighttime sleep. Wherever you are and however you live, traveler or one who is settled down, you can choose to make it an important priority for your life of beauty. In this way, you receive countless benefits both on the inside and consequently permeating through the surface of your body to express itself on the outside. These are the precious priceless hours when the whole body has a chance to repair itself and build anew for you. When you are in the stable environment called home, it's far easier than when you are traveling. It just takes a little planning though, and here's what you do in all those times that you're in other people's homes, hotels, motels, on planes, trains, or anywhere else life takes you. You have small sacred comforting helpers, like a cozy cashmere shawl, an eye pillow and earplugs, a small scented candle, an international time piece to regulate your body, a sleepy time tea bag, your eco friendly re-usable bottle of water filled with your favorite water, and Evian mist for refreshing and hydrating the skin upon waking.

In our society in these trying times it is said we average but a few hours of deep sleep per night, which is why so much advertising focuses on sleep aids of all sorts; and on the repercussions of lack of sleep, like decreased work time due to various disorders of the mind and body; carelessness and exhaustion mid day, hyper alertness at the wrong time of day, mood swings from excess caffeine consumption through a myriad of energy drinks plus the good 'ole cup of coffee or ten that are drunk throughout the day just to stay awake. Imagine if you woke up in the morning happy, refreshed and stretched, yawned and gently in this way welcomed your self to your day. Imagine if you had the energy to wake up just twenty minutes earlier than you used to because now after a couple of months of steady sleep you want to exercise before you even head for the first cup of warm java! Oh, and you're really enjoying that first warm glass of water upon waking to move your bowels and to set the metabolism humming for the rest of the day. Yes, good old -fashioned sleep. A simple decision such as not watching the news an hour before bedtime for a month; or engaging in any heated discussions with your mate, or lengthy listening marathons with girlfriends does wonders for your mind and body in preparation for sleep. Doing nothing other than bathing in the warm cocoon of aromatherapy waters, having sex or gazing gently at uplifting spiritual readings allows the mind to calm, relax and let go. This will prove the kindest most wonderful thing you can do for your appearing and feeling beautiful that I promise your whole life will take on new perspectives if you can really honor this profoundly important ancient secret.

Somehow we develop a relationship to our own beauty by how our light reflects back from the people in our lives. When we, even as children, are welcomed into our families and communities, our own light shines. They welcome us, we welcome the feedback, we again shine our light. Beauty, then, is a positive feedback loop of an energy exchange.

From physics we learn that energy has mass and takes up space. In order for us to create a space or conduit for energy in the body; the body must be open and have flexibility, coordination, balance, strength, and freedom of movement.

Beauty is dynamic and responsive. An attractive man or woman with a self- destructive attitude or habit will detract from their beauty. An attractive person with poor body alignment diminishes their beauty. Clumsiness and rigidity distracts the expression of beauty.

Aesthetically, we can say that a person has a beautiful nose because it is well- shaped and symmetrical. However, a nose by itself can not render beauty until you compare it with other facial features such as the eyes, mouth, and cheekbones. We can see now that beauty can also be a by-product of symmetry, balance, alignment, and movement. Great posture is therefore a vital element of true beauty.

Perhaps we have even witnessed statues which, though inanimate, display symmetry, balance and radiance in color features or posture. Maybe we remember a tree, flower or rock formation that resonates with something inside of us. We feel inspired, comforted, intrigued by this beauty. Nevertheless we are indeed affected in some way.

Again, what appeals to us as beauty has to do with the way light and energy are reflected to the eye of the beholder. The distinguishing human characteristics of beauty are symmetry, movement, character, mind, body and spirit.

Here are some of the indications for great posture and beauty for men and women: Straight toes that have balanced arches. The toes stay straight and centered even through the swing and push-off of a walking stride. The kneecaps are facing forward and the legs are straight (not bowed or knock-knees). The entire pelvis moves in a gyroscopic wave pattern - (Up - Down, Left - Right, Front - Back) to balance the weight of the upper body on its central axis when one is walking. The gyroscopic movement of the pelvis also functions to swing the legs out of each others way during the weight- transfer from Left - to - Right legs and feet.

Special Note Relative To Height and Frame size: A man's pelvis is narrower Left - to - Right, and taller Top - to - Bottom, than a female pelvis. Hence the visual appearance of normal pelvis movement will be considerably more dramatic on a female. A man with the same gyroscopic movement is more likely to be considered "smooth", and not "effeminate". The waist line is perpendicular and level Front - to - Back when viewed from the side, and level Left - to - Right when viewed from the front.

For men and women, the ribcage is open and appears wide at the top, because the arms and shoulders are hanging behind the body's midline. From the back view, the shoulder blades are about one thumb width away from the spine. The top of the chest and the top of the upper back are level Front - to - Back. Mainly for Women: From the side view, the size and weight of the front of the body, (including the front half of the head, the breasts,

torso and thighs) appears to be visually balanced with the weight of the arms and, der-
riere. Actual size and weight do not matter. The
neck appears to lead straight up from the rib
cage to balance head evenly Front - to - Back.
The jawbone is symmetrical Left - to - Right,
in motion

The arms and pelvis swing to balance the
body on a dynamic central axis. When this
occurs, the head appears to be riding in space,
the dynamic dance of great posture is synony-
mous with what makes a person, male or female, beautiful to watch, radiant with
character, charm and personality. Of course,
one is attracted to beauty. It is a natural instinct. It is also a natural instinct to be beautiful, feel happy and feel blessed.

Very often, the realities of living, unfortunately, cause us to distort our natural beauty
and collapse our posture in order to accommo-
date the social, cultural and professional
expectations of others.

This attitude collapse, or the expectation of it, can even occur on a grand scale. How many times have we seen people who are ethnically similar, yet culturally vastly different? Taiwan, Peoples Republic of China, or Chinese American? Barbados, West Africa or Brooklyn? France, Montreal or New Orleans?

Even in a professional or social environment, we may know someone who must express a different aspect of their personality in order to co-exist in that situation. This is not necessarily good or bad. The point is, when one's body is flexible and fully expressive, ones inner beauty comes out.

When our family, culture, and professional expectations give us permission to express our true beauty, then our beauty can be an asset to the entire world. When we can know ourselves thoroughly and accept ourselves confidently, we can be beautiful even if only to ourselves. When our body is flexible and responsive to gravity, size, weight and movement we can have great posture.

A truly beautiful person knows and loves themselves and allows their inner beauty to be an asset to the global community, nation, community, their family, and themselves. All this leads to one point: With great posture you energize your light and let it shine wherever you go. With peace of mind you can allow your body to be free of inhibition and self-doubt.

CHAPTER FIVE

STAY BEAUTIFUL ALL THE TIME

Many modern women place a great deal of importance on physical appearance. Beautiful women are treated much better than average looking women. However, not many women know the secrets to being beautiful. Continue reading to learn more about maximizing your appearance.

Sunglasses can be an accessory that can hurt or help ones beauty. Whether or not someone should wear sunglasses is a decision that is up to the individual in question. Think to yourself "What is the point to these?" " should all be asked.

Improving your appearance begins with your thinking. Most of the differences between people who present themselves positively and those who do not simply comes down to having the right information. Once you know how to take care of yourself it becomes a little less challenging.

Vitamin E is like the Swiss army knife of skin care. It has many different uses. It keeps the skin fresh and smooth looking. Rub a small amount of Vitamin E on your fingernails to alleviate dry, rough cuticles.

Consider using the following beauty tip! Lengthening mascara that is waterproof will make your lashes appear longer and won't run. Many mascaras claim that they can curl your lases and give them more volume. Unfortunately for the consumer, these products are often heavy on the lashes. A heavy mascara could damage your lashes. Only use a formula that is lengthening and waterproof. Your lashes will look thicker and have an upward curl to them.

Beauty tends to focus on skin care quite a bit, but don't neglect your teeth. Being able to deploy a confident, winning smile will serve you well in all your relationships, romantic, friendly, and professional. You will be more successful in what you want to do.

When putting on makeup for work, be minimal. Simply freshen up with foundation and concealer to hide blemishes and maintain a clean look. Use simple, neutral tones for your eye shadow. You can add mascara and eyeliner if you wish. Take care to groom your eyebrows, and don't let them get too out of control. Rather than using a lipstick that dramatically changes your lip color, a more natural look will be achieved with lightly-tinted lip gloss or a lipstick just slightly deeper in shade than your natural tone. Using this technique allows you to look professional and refined throughout the day.

To help keep your skin in good condition, try to use luke-warm water while bathing and showering. Hot water will cause skin pores to expand, and you will lose natural oils your skin needs. These oils are essential to keep your skin moisturized. Use warm or tepid water, as this is more gentle on your skin, keeping it soft and healthy looking. This can also help save money on your water heating costs.

Rubbing a towel on your hair too roughly will damage your hair and make it frizzy. It is better to wrap your hair inside the towel, then pat softly for dryness. Drying your hair this way is slower, but it's much better for it.

Proper sunscreen use is vital to keeping your skin healthy and youthful-looking. Sunscreen isn't only important in the summer; apply sunscreen in winter, as well, to keep wrinkles away. Make sure you apply sunscreen on your faces and hands in the wintertime.

Your follicles will be open and this can cause problems. This can also cause severe irritation to your skin. In the hours after waxing or sugaring, you should stay away from skin care products that contain fragrances. Fragrance can irritate your skin and cause extreme discomfort.

Dab a bit of petroleum jelly on your brows before hitting the hay. Your eyebrows will have a shiny and improved appearance. Don't get the Vaseline anywhere else, though, as it could cause breakouts.

Take a kitchen sponge in your bath and use it to scrub your skin. These work just like a sponge and can be bought in bulk for more savings.

You should never get in the habit of comparing yourself or personal beauty to other people, especially famous people. Since beauty is subjective, what one person finds beautiful the next may not. Try to be happy with you, just the way you are right now.

Avoid rubbing your facial skin. Do this when you are cleaning your face or moisturizing. In addition, don't rub your face during the day, either; when it itches or you are feeling tired. Your skin will look older if you rub it a lot. The best way handle your skin is to lightly pat it, rather than rubbing it.

Use a bit of waterproof mascara if your eyes are feeling tired. This product can open up your eyes and enhance their appearance. Keep extra mascara wands handy so you are able to break clumps up and get rid of flakes around your eyes.

Using a rose or coral colored blush can help to soften your look, especially if you have a sharper square shaped face. Use your fingers to apply the cream to your cheeks. Next, use a gentle, pulling motion to blend the color up towards your temples.

If you are going to blow dry your hair, be sure to use a heat protection spray beforehand in order to prevent damage. You can find this in generic stores. It's used to prevent split ends and help your hair dry *q*uicker. It smells great and helps your hair retain moisture.

If you want to have soft feet, use petroleum jelly. Coconut oil is a reasonably priced, all natural oil that soaks in clean and softens skin deeply. Rubbing it on your feet every other day will keep them soft and smooth.

Try putting Vaseline on your heels and feet while you sleep. Your feet will be soft and smooth like they are after a pedicure. Using this techni*q*ue routinely every single night will ensure you don't forget to do it. After applying the vaseline, take out a pair of socks and cover your feet before going to sleep.

CHAPTER SIX

ULTIMATE BEAUTY SECRETS

We've all experienced a fashion emergency or wished we could improve out beauty regimen with easy, inexpensive adjustments. So here are some *q*uick and easy ways to stave off that unsightly pimple, keep under eye bags at bay and have gorgeous skin all year long.

Pimple Rx

Feel a pimple coming on and can't walk around with chalky white toothpaste on your face? Try dabbing some of your perfume on the blemish a few times throughout the day. The alcohol in the perfume will help dry it out (plus you'll smell great!).

Sleep better

Have trouble falling asleep but you've exhausted your sleep aid prescription? Why not try to catch some Z's the natural way? Lavender is known to promote alpha waves, which are necessary for restful sleep. Try soaking in a bath before bed with Lavender salts or Lavender oil.

Here's another idea: take a Lavender face pillow and pop it in the microwave on low for a couple of minutes, then place inside your pillowcase. Put your arms over your head and clasp hands, then stretch your clasped arms as far to the right as possible (make sure you remain comfortable) and then back over your body to the left. Repeat about five times.

Breathe in deeply as you do these stretches, which will get the oxygen flowing.

Perfect that Pout

We can only dream of having lips like Angelina-well naturally anyway. Most of us have at least thought about using a lip plumper, hoping to look in the mirror and see gloriously luscious lips smiling back at us. The key is getting lips ready for lip plumper, so it can penetrate and do its job.

Here's a little trick that won't cost you a dime. Apply a small amount of Vaseline on a soft bristle tooth brush that's been moistioned with warm water. Ever so gently brush lips for about 2 minutes-you might want to do this while watching TV, two minutes can feel like forever. Remove the Vaseline with moistened towelette or soft washcloth and then blot dry. Apply moisturizer, sunscreen and lip plumper.

Then go show off your beautifully plumped lips.

P.S. If you don't want to splurge on a store-bought lip plumper, dab a tiny-and we mean tiny-amount of Cayenne pepper on your lips. It'll sting a little, but what's a little pain in the name of looking gorgeous?

Baby Soft Skin

Wonder why some women appear to have plump, hydrated skin even in the middle of winter while yours is so dry it hurts to smile? Chances are those other ladies are doing a few things differently-or else they are genetically perfect and we don't like them anyway.

When it comes to keeping your skin hydrated it only makes sense to drink lots of water. Water keeps the cells in your body quenched, so your skin looks luminous and your appetite is curbed (great skin and a trim figure-it's too for the price of one!). You've is-especially if you don't have a $200 a month beauty budget-is that you can still yourself to radiant, glowing skin for the cost of your daily Starbucks and muffin, just by visiting your local drugstore. There are lots of great moisurizers that hydrate and condition dry, thirsty skin with natural ingredients like shea butter and vitamin E.

In addition to applying lotion daily, here are some other helpful tips to keep skin smooth during the winter months:

Keep your shower times shorter and limit your exposure to hot water. Try turning on the radio and limiting yourself to just 2-3 songs as a guide.

Avoid intense scrubbing while showering. Choose a soft soap rather than an exfolient. Here's an idea. The Beauty Skin Cloth gently exfoliates the skin with a special texture that stimulates blood circulation, while requiring you to use less soap.

Don't forget your sunscreen! Sun damage

can still happen with clouds in the sky, so it's very important to continue to wear no less than SPF 15 every day.

Frizz-free hair

On the go and forgot your hair pomade? Don't freak out-and certainly don't let your hair freak out. Apply a small dollup of hand lotion in your hands, then gently smooth hands over your hair. This will help to tame unruly hair. You can also use a tiny amount of Vaseline on the ends of your hair.

De-puff eyes

Computer strain, too little sleep, too much sleep, stress-you name it and it can makes your eyes puff up like a cream cheese wonton. If you're looking for a quick fix that's more effective than cucumbers, try a green tea or black tea bag (it must contain caffeine). Dip it in hot water then toss it in the freezer for 5 minutes. If you have some foresight pop an anti-histamine like Benedryl the night before and you'll wake up bag-free. Supplements can help with puffiness too. MSM with Glucosamine, Flax Oil and Evening Primrose Oil seem to help alleviate puffiness.

Fake tan streaks

With all the publicity about skin cancer you feel guilty getting a tan the old fashioned way. So you tried a self-tanner or maybe you opted for the Mystic Tan booth. Unfortunately you ended up with the telltale streaks on your arms, legs, feet ... okay everywhere. Don't worry, you don't have to wear a turtleneck and pants until it fades. Hop in the shower right away (some will inevitably come off anyway) and generously rub down with an exfoliating body scrub followed by a rigorous scrubbing with a loofah. For really bad cases around the ankles, feet, elbows and hands (usually the driest parts of your body), you can use a callous file to eliminate unsightly streaks. We don't recommend incorporating these measures into your regular routine but if you've got a big event you can't exactly show up looking like you got in a fight with a can of orange spray paint either.

Better yet--avoid rubbing your skin raw with St. Tropez Self-Tan Remover. Like magic it removes unsightly stains from your palms and other body parts if you mess up (the only caveat: it only works up to 4 hours after you apply self tanner). Find it at Sephora, Bath and Body Works, Victoria's Secret and Red Door Salons.

For a more even self-tanner application, try Tan Airbrush in a Can.

When You Don't Have ...

Hair Gel USE ... Lotion

heard it before but we'll say it again, get eight 8oz glasses a day. Your skin will thank you.

Here's something you may not have heard before: distilled water is the best for drinking because chlorine and other contaminants are greatly reduced when the water is boiled. To hydrate your skin throughout the day try a purified water mister.

Moisturizing Basics

The best time to moisturize is immediately after bathing when your body is damp and moist. Smooth on Body Butter, Body Cream, or Body Lotion to lock in moisture. And you don't have to spend a lot of money.

Some may think the more expensive a moisturizer is, the more effective it will be against dry skin. But this really is a myth. That's not to say expensive lotions don't make us feel more luxurious (even if it's just because we know how much it cost). But the good news

Mascara USE ... Vaseline (It Works! Just Go Light, You Don't Want To Have Gloppy Lashes)

Zit Cream USE ... Perfume For On-The-Go/White Toothepaste For At-Home Use Only.

Lip Gloss USE ... Vaseline

Neosporan USE ... Honey

Lip Plumper USE ... Cayenne Pepper

Eye Gel USE ... Frozen Tea Bags

CHAPTER SEVEN

DOES BEAUTY CAUSE JEALOUSY?

Women can be so beastly to one another. Women can also be the perpetrators of hate towards other women. Women can instigate and continue a trail of destruction towards another woman.

It can be very uncomfortable to acknowledge that women can act just as aggressively as men and cause the emotional breakdown in others especially towards other women.

There are many diverse and oddly strange

reasons for women behaving badly and jealousy is one of those reasons.

When the green eye of envy glares from the pulpit of internal vision in a woman, the results can range from mild verbal contact to being downright unbelievably heinous. Due to jealousy, a woman could temporarily appear insane. Some behaviours include verbal rages appearing irrational and incessant; her stiffened body taut from the venom squeezing from every pore. Jealousy is potent and can destroy both the holder and the receiver.

The Beauty Myth looks at the overall impact on women and we will be examining the psychological impact on women. To surmise the concept and explain the Beauty Myth, here is a quick précis.

The Beauty Myth is an allegorical ideology about what a woman should look like to be readily accepted in society. Men, for control over women construct this ideology. The ideology of beauty as in the Beauty Myth is not defined, therefore there are no clear guidelines or demarcation.

There are many ways in which a woman gravitates towards making herself appealing and to appease men and the resulting language, spoken or not, determines how women view themselves. Women then systematically enshrine the essence of the Beauty Myth by plundering themselves to a regime of incessant grooming including the use of surgery, cosmetics and diets. A woman does not have to be aware of the Beauty Myth to be complicit in its language. The control over women by men renders women out of control in mind and body as she strives for attainment of acceptance. Remember, what the actual concept of beauty should look like is not defined! Whilst this is happening locally for women, the woman then sees other women as potential rivals. Women compete with other women vying for the attention from men creating a war on each other that may appear

comical to some but is in no doubt very debil-
itating for women reciprocally.

Women readily accept striving to achieve
the 'ideal' weight and maintain this notion even
at the risk of their own health. In some con-
texts, this ideal is nothing short of experimenting with their life. In an attempt to mask
over her own lack of self-esteem, a woman
may originate a furtive competition with her
colleagues, peers and even friends to appear to
be the better looking therefore more acceptable
to men. Is the archetypal jealous woman real or
fictitious? Just take a look around you.

Women eyeing up other women whilst
measuring their own selves and sometimes
leaving others feeling as though they are below
standard. If a particular woman measures
against another woman and feels she is more
attractive than she perceives her 'rival' to be,
just watch her physiology prolifically change
in an instant. If she perceives this same 'rival'
to be featuring an attribute she is keen to

personally gain this same change in her physiology is evident but this time, she retreats within herself. The Omni-presence of the Beauty Myth is indeed powerful even if not understood by its participants. The concept of the Beauty Myth makes women jealous towards other women a certainty.

Young girls are tenacious; they are determined and self-assured. They can appear bossy and knows how to get their wishes completed. They can manipulate others for their gains without blinking. The young female knows who she is and will fight for control in her circle. (This description is architypically of young females before society teaches them that their voices are not to be heard, another discussion!) Many times, the young female who views herself as mentally and emotionally strong will seek friends who appear to her to be the opposite of her traits. This way, she will continue to reign. When she does befriend another young female who then goes on to outwardly presenting with the same strong traits, they may remain friends but will experience bouts of rivalry towards each other. However, why they would remain as friends needs further explaining. The need to reign is secondary in spiritual terms to the more important aspect of having, nurturing and maintaining friends. This means that whilst the need to reign is strong, this is borne from the pressures put on them from their outside world. The need for friends is borne from their inner world (subconscious) and is much stronger than the need to reign. Young females, growing females and grown females will find a comfortable place with each other that accommodates their rivalry as long as they are friends. So does this mean that the Beauty Myth perpetuates the traits already found in females and uses it against them?

The competition between women to beautify self to surpass their 'rival' is not done explicitly. There are no words that are used that determine such acts of rivalry; the competition is clandestine. There are times when a female will depict her sense of being at war when she negatively calls on the 'flaw' of her rival, teasing her about her perceived 'afflictions.' Or when a female has been perceived to have 'achieved' the mythological beauty, the backlash from her peers is all too evident. The sniping, the backbiting or even the silent treatments towards to the poor female are tools that are used to demonstrate the discomfort women feel towards their 'rival' but borne from their own lack of a positive self identity. The need to reign (starting in early age) is ever-present but made more complex when they become older and now also vying for acceptance from men.

Young girls in the playground demonstrably sending some other poor girl 'out to Coventry' merely for having a super pair of shiny shoes that the reigning girl does not. The teenage female who turns on her friend because that boy she likes is not reciprocal with her attention-seeking activities. The new woman at work who makes the standardised corporate uniform look incredibly perceptively sexy even without trying. Supermodels are dicing with their health in an attempt to be the thinnest therefore prettiest amongst her peers. She has learnt that this ensures continuous work for her. Media depict background scenes of the clichéd females behaving beastly towards each other in the same attempt to reign and be accepted. Movie celebrities all seeking the reduced weight as the camera 'puts on pounds' and media shouts out any imperfections on a woman in a public way. Not all publicity is good publicity! Feuds are started by women with other women just because of perceptions based on looks. Especially worsened if the female celebrity is newsworthy and overexposed. So all women are somehow affected by beauty and can become, coupled with a typically feminine trait, extend into jealousy. The levels to which jealously can extend to, is dependent upon what the attacking female feels she has to gain to extinguish her rival or equally how she much she has to lose.

Here are a few explanations of jealousy:

Fearful or wary of being supplanted; apprehensive of losing affection or position; resentment or bitter in rivalry; having to do with or arising from feelings of envy, apprehension or bitterness; vigilant in guarding something; intolerant of disloyalty or infidelity, autocratic.

The need to feel beautiful therefore accepted by self and others is inextricably linked to having better self-esteem. This increases the competition in and for women. The 'rewards' are both self-serving to women and for men. However, with the Omni-presence of the Beauty Myth makes jealously a sure fire win for men, whoever wins the competition, they cannot lose. Until women build their self-esteem on feelings on individualism, compassion for other women and acceptance of other women and their equally beautiful features, the war with jealousy will continue. The Beauty Myth continues to reign over the female who thinks she reigns. Until women understand that they are men's half-witted sense of delusions and will never aspire to true equality, they remain incarcerated spiritually. The creation of 'the woman' needs to happen and how this is done is by understanding who they are and remove self from men's expectation. Women then need to build up spiritually by becoming aware of their inner resources to begin the trade off with men for equality because at the moment, men do not have to trade with women on equal grounds.

BEAUTY TIPS FOR WOMEN TO STAY HEALTHY AND BEAUTIFUL

Beauty tips for women is an ongoing search, and one great temptations, if you can afford it, is to use surgery to help cover up your natural aging. Sadly, there are many reports from women who feel that they now look worse after their expensive plastic surgery than they did before. Rather than taking a chance of an operation gone wrong, there are lots of tips and techniques that you can use to keep yourself looking and feeling beautiful rather than opting for an operation. In this article we will examine some beauty tips that will allow you to wear your age with pride and confidence.

Diet

Diet is perhaps one of the most important beauty tips for women towards having and maintaining a healthy look. Consuming lots of fruits, vegetables and protein-rich foods does more than just benefit your general health. A diet like this also helps to prevent weight gain and increases your energy levels to keep you active during your day. These types of foods also have the benefits of encouraging strong healthy and shiny hair, strong fingernails, and results skin that has a healthy radiance.

Water

Never underestimate the importance of drinking enough water daily which makes it one of the top beauty tips for women. There are numerous benefits of avoiding dehydration, one of them being the effect it has on the appearance of your skin tone. Many common beverages such as pop, coffee and especially alcohol actually help to dry out your skin and encourage the growth of wrinkles. To avoid these dehydrating effects that may lead to wrinkles, it is important to drink lots of water and use a daily moisturizer. A simple but effective combination to reduce the occurrence of wrinkles. Smokers and sun worshippers also run the risk of seeing premature wrinkles, so it is essential that sun screen be worn on hot summer days, even when cloudy. Giving up smoking will not only discourage wrinkles, but may allow you to live longer as well.

Regular Exercise

Any listing of beauty tips for women would

not be complete without mentioning the need and importance of regular exercise to maintain good health and good looks as we all age. Keeping active is the key, whether you enjoy simply walking or more strenuous activities such as jogging, swimming, cycling or sports such as soccer, hockey, baseball, tennis, skiing, and the list goes on and on. All of these activities will help to keep you healthy and feeling good about yourself so that you will not even consider any type of surgery to deal with aging. Another spin-off of regular exercise is the hidden benefit it also has on your mental state and how you feel about yourself.

Age Acceptance

Our final point in beauty tips for women is all about age acceptance. Learning to live with their age is something that many people refuse to accept. Often this age denial results in these people making complete fools of themselves in public! As an example, women in their 50s trying to dress like 20-year olds wearing tight clothing and bleached hair, when clearly they do not have the figure or appearance to pull it off. Certainly not one of the beauty tips that we want to encourage!

Instead learn to dress and behave in ways that are expected for people your age. Embrace your age and looks rather than trying to be someone you obviously are not, at least not for the past 20 years. This is not to say that there is anything wrong with wearing fashionable or trendy clothes or for that matter dying your hair to cover up the grey, but don't end up looking like a clown in the process! You can look and feel young at heart without being the centre of attention for the wrong reasons.

Aging is a natural process that everyone must deal with. Sadly many people refuse to accept this fact and rather than learning to live with it and look at the positives, they spend their days, and sometimes large sums of money, trying to cheat nature. Rather than searching online and reading book after book on beauty tips and looking for the magic pill for eternal youth they should pay attention to the basics.

Simply eat healthy foods, drink lots of water, engage in a regular exercise routine and learn how to be beautiful by following these basic beauty tips for women. This will help you to look and feel great about your current age, whatever it is now, and will be in the future.

CHAPTER EIGHT

BEAUTY TIPS FOR WOMEN OVER 50

Women over 50 need to take care of their beauty to look younger and beautiful. They are required to pay special attention to care their skin and can delay aging for the time being. They should use creamy lipsticks rather than a gloss or matte to look beautiful. You can either use a lip balm that should contain vitamin E or you can also apply Vaseline to look good.

There is no reason for it that why women don't look beautiful after 50. It is impossible to stop aging forever, but you can preserve your youthful looks for many years to come, ward off wrinkles and keep your skin softer.

There are some tips which makes the women look beautiful in the age of 50

· As you get older, you tend to dehydrate and your skin gets dryer. Drinking plenty of water will help your skin hydrated from the inside out of your body.

- You need to take good nutrition to repair skin from damaging. It must include all the nutrients that help to stay fit and younger.
- You are recommended to start exercise to improve your physical condition. These exercises increase your flexibility, reduce depression and even improve memory. This will help you to stay fit and beautiful at age of 50.
- Do not use soaps that makes the

skin dryer. Use moisturizing soaps and lotions to avoid aging.

- Applying a face mask in a month will leave your skin smooth and wrinkle-free. You must apply to the back of your hands and leave it for 15-20 minutes as hands can also reveal you age.

- You must use sunscreen with spf of 15 to protect your skin from UVB and UVA radicals.

- You can even apply heavy make-up and powders to your skin which will make it dry and matte and choose a lip liner which helps you to define lips.

CHAPTER NINE

BEAUTY IDEAS FOR WOMEN

A woman wants to look beautiful all her life and a beautiful you will come with boosted confidence and a high self-esteem. It is important to know the best ways to take care of your skin, hair, eyes and nails in order to remain beautiful. Among the beauty tips for women is a lifestyle change that involves a healthy diet and healthy habits. The skin responds to what we eat and a healthy looking skin indicates a healthy diet. Eating a balanced diet is necessary and the skin will flourish in diets that are high on fruits and vegetables. These help in replenishing the skin to give it a healthy glow. Taking up to eight glasses of water daily is another beauty tip that will ensure that your skin is well cleansed.

To keep that skin glowing, it is advisable to embark on the three-phase treatment for the face that includes cleansing, toning and moisturizing. The first thing you do is to wash your face with the appropriate face wash, which is followed by cleansing. Toning comes third followed with moisturizing which ensures that your face does not dry up. Using a sunscreen is highly recommended at all times since the skin is very sensitive to weather changes. Overexposure to sun is a known cause for skin cancers and it is therefore important to ensure that you wear your sunscreen in all weather. The lips are a prominent feature on the face and you do not want to walk around with dry chipped lips. It is therefore best to apply lip balm, Vaseline or a petroleum jelly to ensure that they are well moisturized through the day. Hair defines a woman and the healthier it looks the better.

Among the beauty tips for women is trimming your hair often to rid it of split ends. It is also advisable to keep it healthy using henna packs, natural proteins or amla-reetha-shikakai packs. Hair must be kept moisturized and oils such as almond, castor, and olive are highly recommended. To ensure that your scalp stays clean and dandruff free, it is important to shampoo your hair at least twice a week. Conditioning it is vital, as it will ensure that it is soft and manageable. Styling your hair appropriately makes up the beauty tips for women and it is important to style it according to your face shape. Another beauty tip for women is indulging in a body massage weekly to ensure that your body stays firm and hydrated.

To remove the unwanted hair, it is ideal to opt for waxing for the legs and hands. When buying cosmetics, it is important to test them to ensure that they do not end up harming your skin. This is done through a patch test to ensure that it does not react with your skin or cause allergic conditions. Beauty tips for women on cosmetics insist that you should stick to one brand that works for your skin since experimentation with many others may make your skin sensitive. Another important beauty tip is to ensure that you remove your entire make up before retiring to bed. This ensures that you do not take debris to bed, which may cause rashes, acne, and excessive oil secretions.

CHAPTER TEN

BEAUTY TIPS FOR WOMEN OVER 60

As you get older, only then can you perceive your real beauty. Women, in the period they grow older and age - they crave to look beautiful as everything requires a special attention. Beauty tips for women over 60 encourage taking care of your hairstyle, erasing off the aging marks, wrinkles, and use makeup accordingly so that your appearance does not look false.

You dressing sense, boasting of a beautiful skin, taking proper care to boast a lovely body and possessing a brilliant styling sense - nothing should stop although you may have hit the 60s. The most important factor is that you need to follow an extremely balanced and proper diet and skin care. Skin care is as much about what goes in your body as it is about what you apply to the surface. Therefore, unless you nourish your body from inside, there is no way you can seek healthy and glowing skin. Make sure you eat a proper diet comprised of fresh vegetables, fresh fruits and whole grains.

As you grow older, you should increase the intake of Vitamin A and Vitamin E enriched foods. This is to replenish the natural amounts of vitamins within the body. Vitamin A and Vitamin E promote new cell growth within the skin surface and make it appear more radiant. This is essential for the natural cell regeneration process of the body.

So make sure you eat lots of green and yellow vegetables! As we age, our skin loses moisture and becomes dry and tight. It develops a wrinkled texture and appears dull and lifeless. This dryness is caused by the hormonal changes, loss of moisture from the upper layers of the skin and a decrease in intracellular lipids. Always remember to moisturize your skin properly.

1. Here Are Some Simple Beauty Tips for Women over 60:
2. Work with a cream lipstick instead of a matte or gloss
3. Work with a neutral lip liner as that will add plumpness to it
4. A lip liner can be used to define the lips
5. The lip liner color should be very close to the natural shade of your lips
6. You could carry the different lipstick shades (all in daring colors) to fit different occasions, outfits, and moods.

7. Avoid the use of heavy makeup
8. Avoid the use of too much of powder as it will only make your skin more dry and give a matte look.
9. Use moisturizing soaps and lotions to hydrate your skin.
10. Your diet should be proper and balanced
11. Drinking plenty of water will help you to hydrate the skin
12. SPF 15 or higher products should be used with both UVB and UVA protection.
13. Simple Tips of Beauty for Women over 60
14. Have confidence in the fact that you are beautiful and it is always advisable to look beautiful from inside
15. Know your individual personality

and spice up and sport your identity accordingly

16. Match your attire with the perfect pair of shoes.
17. Use colors - be it in case of makeup, dresses and accessories
18. Laugh and you will then find a natural glow on your face.

You don't have to always be judgmental, just try out experimenting new exciting things. The world has definitely changed a lot over the years, but it is okay to change with it.

CHAPTER ELEVEN

WOMAN HEALTH AND BEAUTY TIPS

Being a woman is more than having feminine organs, is learning to understand your body at different stages of life and anticipate the small ailments before they become real problems. Your body's needs when you were a 17-year-old girl cannot be the same as when you are a 57 year old. However, no matter your age, at one time or another, being women, your health and beauty will be affected by one of the following conditions: facial wrinkles, virginal infection, abnormal menstruation, breast drooping, women infertility, cellulite, stretch marks, spider vein, varicose vein, menopause, Constipation, depression, vitamin deficiency, and the list goes on.

How to Have Healthy, Beautiful Skin?

Every woman wants to have a radiant skin; unfortunately, most of them don't figure out the causes of their skin problems. Each day, our body is attacked by pollution, the sun, sweat, stress, abuse of all kinds such as tobacco, alcohol and unhealthy fast foods. To have a healthy, beautiful skin, it is important to reverse the effects of those aggressors by adopting a healthy lifestyle including eating a healthy diet regular exercise, and good sleep.

However, sometimes, all these efforts on a daily basis are not enough. The more we advance in age, the more the body requires small attentions that require a little cosmetic. We advice you to use safe and natural skin products.

Safe and natural products, applied regularly, can help greatly to protect your look from the ravages of time and pollution. Feminine beauty to please men and make you feel good about yourself. Finding yourself beautiful is essential to live in harmony with yourself and others.

Keep your skin clean and clear. Taking care of yourself is taking care of your skin on a daily basis. Cleaning the skin must be made daily using products that do not alter its natural balance or damage it. The skin is exposed to external aggression. By its peripheral position, the skin is unavoidably attacked by dust, pollution, which mingling to the sebum and sweat disrupt the balance of its surface. You need natural antioxidant cream to repair those damages. Today, unconsciously, people tend to excessive use of gels or anti-aging products that are, most of times, do more harm to the skin. Be aware that those products can increase your skin's risk of UV damage.

. . .

Taking care of your face

Your face is your passport; do not ever neglect it. The skin of your face is constantly assaulted by the environment: temperature too high or too low, wind, pollution, temperature changes. It needs to be protected by the use of an anti-oxidant cream. Protective cream or restorative cream, the choice of your cream depends on your skin type and your needs. Living in cities, cold, working outdoors or in a confined place, your cream facial must also provide a degree of protection that suits your lifestyle. It must also be adapted to the nature of your skin (dry skin, oily skin, mixed skin), the choice of your moisturizer is essential to better protect the skin of your face and allow it to find the right balance.

Femininity of a beautiful neckline

The arms and chest areas are very sensitive and are also a sign of femininity that each of us likes to discover. But often, the years pass, with a few kilos too many, and not enough physical activity, mean that our arms, our breasts are no longer as energetic as before and become a real complex. These areas are very fragile because they do not have true muscle support and are therefore subject to rapid aging, wrinkles, skin falling and flaccid. For, too often, the neck and chest are forgotten in the care of daily hydration. However, they must be washed, hydrated and treated the same way as the face.

To preserve the elasticity of the skin of those areas, it is important to apply every morning a nourishing and moisturizing cream, taking care to apply a light massage that will activate the superficial microcirculation. Apply a special cream by massaging lightly and gently from the center of the breast to cover the entire breast and up to the neck.

. . .

Intimate hygiene

Often taboo, the subject of personal hygiene is often not discussed despite the great importance it takes. What are the gestures to comply, products to use, learn all relevant information. Because staying fresh is a daily concern for both well-being and health, intimate hygiene should not be overlooked. Be simple and natural in your virginal care; any negligence or overuse of chemical can lead to vaginal issues. In a relationship, vaginal odor is a tough problem for both partners. It is embarrassing for the female, and frustrating for the male.

What products to use for personal hygiene?

All products, shower gels, soaps and bubble baths variety are not necessarily suited for intimate hygiene. Often too aggressive, their pH (acidity level) is different from that of our skin and does not respect the natural balance. The acidity of genital mucous makes it possible to ensure the maintenance of vulvo-virginal flora necessary to preserve the female genitals of fungal infections and diverse.

Hygiene and menstruation

Whether you use tampons or pads, change them regularly, about every 4 hours (except at night where you can keep them until morning). If you use tampons, be sure to choose the model adapted to the flow of your menstruation, which also varies between the beginning and the end of your period. A tampon too big and absorbing, at the end of the cycle, can irritate the vagina and lead the development of a fungus. In the same way, a tampon changed too frequently can be a source of irritation.

Healthy and beautiful legs

Take care of your legs. The legs are one of the female assets, but can also be a source of much inconvenience. Those who have heavy legs, varicose veins or Restless legs syndrome. If you want to attract men, pay attention to your legs, they say. Most men get turned on by a hot woman's legs. Men love looking at women's hot, sexy legs; maybe there is a secret in that.

What could affect the beauty and health of your legs? - High heels, consumption of alcohol and cigarettes and an unbalanced diet are all aggravating factors of poor blood circulation and therefore pain in the legs with obviously appearance of cellulite, stretch marks and small vessels that burst.

Advice to have beautiful and healthy legs - The fundamental solution is regular exercises with more precisely jogging and jumping. The legs acquire, through regular exercises, greater finesse and elasticity. Their muscles develop harmoniously and the entire body usually takes profits with improved blood circulation.

Diet

Numerous researchers confirm that a healthy nutrition makes a positive difference in skin rejuvenation. Your beauty has a close relationship with what you eat. You are what you eat, they say. However, even if you eat a healthy diet, you also need to avoid eating late at night. Do your best to eat at least 3 hours before going to bed. Eating late can cause chronic indigestion, which can lead to acne, bad breath, belly fat, eczema, and psoriasis. Adjust your diet to your life (sedentary lifestyle, active, sportive), your condition (pregnant, obeses), your age (children, youth, adult, elderly) in order not to create imbalance in your diet. Energy needs vary depending on sex and a multitude of other factors.

The feminine beauty perfect is "the socially constructed perception that bodily splendor is certainly one of ladies's maximum essential belongings, and something all women have to try to obtain and maintain. female splendor beliefs are rooted in heteronormative ideals, and closely affect women of all sexual orientations. The feminine beauty ideal, which also includes lady body shape, varies from culture to lifestyle. strain to conform to a sure definition of "stunning" may have drastic mental effects. those ideals had been correlated with depression, consuming issues, and low shallowness, starting from a teenager age and persevering with into adulthood.

www.ingramcontent.com/pod-product-compliance
Lightning Source LLC
Chambersburg PA
CBHW031133020426
42333CB00012B/352